LIGHT THERAPY

Complete Guide To Harnessing The Healing Power Of Light Therapy For Optimal Wellness And Radiant Health

WILFREDO CARSON

INTRODUCTION

Light therapy, often known as phototherapy, is a medical treatment that uses precise wavelengths of light to treat a variety of illnesses. It has gained popularity in recent years due to its therapeutic applications in a wide spectrum of medical and psychiatric conditions. Light therapy has a long history, dating back to ancient civilizations when sunshine was recognized for its restorative powers. Over time, technological developments have enabled more targeted and controlled use of light in medical settings. This chapter presents an overview of light therapy, including its definition, historical background, importance, scope, and the book's objectives.

1.1 Definition of Light Therapy.

Light therapy is the employment of specific wavelengths of light to induce biological responses within the body for therapeutic purposes. The light used in this treatment is generally brilliant and resembles natural sunlight. It is administered via light boxes, lamps, or other devices that deliver the necessary intensity and spectrum of light. Light therapy's therapeutic effects are linked to its influence on circadian rhythm, neurotransmitters, and different physiological systems. As a growing subject, the concept of light therapy expands as researchers investigate new uses and improve old methods.

1.2 Historical Background:

Light treatment originated in ancient civilizations, where sunshine was respected for its therapeutic effects.

The Ancient Greeks, Egyptians, and Romans recognized the medicinal effects of sunlight and incorporated it into their medical methods. The Danish doctor Niels Rydberg Finsen received the Nobel Prize in Physiology or Medicine in the early twentieth century for his work on light therapy in disease treatment, particularly lupus. The invention of artificial light sources in the mid-twentieth century paved the path for more precise and focused light treatment. Since then, research has expanded to include applications in dermatology, psychology, and neurology.

1.3 Significance and Scope of Light Therapy:

Light therapy is important in modern healthcare because of its numerous applications and non-invasive nature. One of its principal applications is the treatment of seasonal affective disorder (SAD), a type of depression that occurs at specific periods of the year, typically in the fall and winter when sunshine exposure is limited. Aside from psychiatric problems, light therapy has been useful in the treatment of dermatological conditions such as psoriasis and dermatitis. Furthermore, continuing research is investigating its potential in treating sleep problems, circadian rhythm disruptions, and potentially certain neurological illnesses.

The breadth of light therapy extends beyond traditional medical settings, including applications in sports medicine and performance enhancement. Athletes employ light therapy to boost recovery and performance by altering elements including sleep quality and muscle regeneration. Furthermore, light therapy is being investigated as a supplemental treatment for disorders such as chronic pain, where its analgesic effects may provide respite to people who suffer from constant discomfort.

1.4 Goals of the Book:

The goal of this book is to provide a thorough understanding of light therapy, its mechanisms of action, and its applications in a variety of medical fields. The book attempts to investigate the most recent research discoveries, technical breakthroughs, and emerging trends in the field. It aims to be a beneficial resource for healthcare professionals, researchers, and students who want to learn more about the science of light therapy and its potential impact on human health and well-being. Each chapter focuses on a unique component of light therapy, ranging from the fundamental physiological processes to practical issues for execution.

In later chapters, we will look at the physiological principles by which light therapy works, the specific applications in many medical sectors, and the ongoing research that is shaping the ever-changing landscape of this therapeutic modality.

This book intends to contribute to the knowledge base by providing a thorough examination of light therapy's potential benefits and limitations in the field of healthcare.

CHAPTER 1
FUNDAMENTALS OF LIGHT

Light is a type of electromagnetic radiation perceptible to the human eye. It has a significant impact on many elements of life, including human health. Understanding the fundamental properties of light is critical for pursuing therapeutic uses.

Properties of Light

Wavelengths and frequencies are essential properties that characterize the nature of light. Wavelength is the distance between successive peaks or troughs in a wave, whereas frequency is the number of oscillations per unit of time. In the context of light treatment, different wavelengths are connected with varied therapeutic effects.

Longer wavelengths, such as those in the red and infrared spectrums, are known to penetrate deeper into tissues, making them ideal for some therapeutic uses. Shorter wavelengths, such as those in the blue spectrum, offer antibacterial qualities and are used to treat various skin problems.

Photons, the fundamental particles of light, convey energy in proportion to their frequency. Understanding photon behavior is critical for understanding the mechanisms underlying light therapy. The electromagnetic spectrum includes all types of electromagnetic radiation, including as radio waves, microwaves, infrared radiation, visible light, ultraviolet radiation, X-rays, and gamma rays. Each part of this spectrum has distinct features and interactions with biological tissues, which serve as the foundation for a variety of light therapy therapeutic options.

The Function of Light in Human Health.

The role of light in human health goes beyond its visual function. Light affects the circadian rhythm, a natural, endogenous process that regulates the sleep-wake cycle and occurs approximately every 24 hours. The circadian cycle is sensitive to light, specifically fluctuations in intensity and color temperature. Exposure to natural light during the day, particularly in the morning, helps regulate the circadian cycle, resulting in greater sleep and overall well-being. Circadian rhythm disruptions, which are frequently caused by insufficient exposure to natural light, inconsistent sleep patterns, or nighttime exposure to artificial light, have been related to a variety of health problems, including sleep difficulties, mood abnormalities, and reduced immune function.

Furthermore, light aids in the creation of vitamin D in the skin. Sunlight's ultraviolet B (UVB) radiation triggers the formation of vitamin D, which is essential for bone health, immunological function, and overall well-being. Adequate exposure to natural light is therefore required to maintain appropriate vitamin D levels in the body.

<u>Natural Sources of Light</u>

The sun is the primary naturally occurring source of light. Solar radiation has a wide range of wavelengths, providing a variety of therapeutic benefits. Sunlight exposure is important not just for vitamin D synthesis, but also for circadian rhythm regulation and mental health promotion. Different times of day provide varying intensities and colors of light, which influence the body's physiological responses.

Morning sunshine, which is rich in blue wavelengths, promotes awake and alertness, whereas evening sunlight's warmer tones tell the body to prepare for sleep.

Natural light is more than just a source of illumination; it is also a complex stimulus that regulates hormones, neurotransmitters, and other biochemical processes in the body. According to research, exposure to natural light improves mood, cognitive function, and overall mental wellness. Incorporating natural light into the built environment, such as using daylighting in architectural design, has become a priority for improving occupant well-being in a variety of situations.

<u>Artificial Light Sources</u>

Artificial light sources have become an essential aspect of modern living, providing illumination in indoor settings and extending the availability of light beyond daylight hours. However, not all artificial light sources are the same, and their effects on human health differ. Incandescent, fluorescent, LED and other lighting technologies produce light of varying spectrum compositions, color temperatures, and intensities.

The color temperature of artificial light, measured in kelvins (K), affects its biological effects. Cooler light with higher color temperatures, similar to sunshine, has been connected with better attentiveness and performance. Warmer light with lower color temperatures, such as evening sunshine, promotes relaxation and sleep. The use of artificial lighting in a variety of settings, including homes, workplaces, and healthcare facilities, can have a major impact on persons' well-being and productivity.

In recent years, there has been an increased interest in the development of light sources specifically designed for therapeutic purposes. Light-emitting diodes (LEDs) are popular in light treatment devices because of their ability to emit precise wavelengths of light. These devices, which range from handhelds for localized treatments to bigger panels for whole-body exposure, are utilized for several therapeutic purposes, including skin rejuvenation, pain management, and mood modulation.

Understanding the interaction between natural and artificial light sources is critical for maximizing the advantages of light therapy. Balancing exposure to natural light with the strategic use of artificial light sources can help to maintain a healthy circadian rhythm, promote psychological well-being, and utilize light's therapeutic potential in a variety of medical procedures.

Studying the principles of light gives a good foundation for understanding its diverse significance in human health. Understanding the fundamental qualities of light and its various sources, both natural and artificial, is critical for unlocking the therapeutic potential of light in the developing discipline of light therapy. As researchers continue to uncover the intricate mechanisms underlying light's impact on the human body, incorporating light therapy into healthcare procedures shows promise for boosting overall well-being.

CHAPTER 2
BIOLOGICAL EFFECTS OF LIGHT

Circadian rhythms:

Circadian rhythms are biological cycles that regulate many physiological and behavioral processes in living organisms. The term "circadian" is derived from the Latin words "circa" (meaning "around") and "diem" (meaning "day"), emphasizing the approximately 24-hour cycle of these rhythms. Understanding the body's internal clock is critical for appreciating the complex systems that regulate circadian rhythms.

The suprachiasmatic nucleus (SCN) of the hypothalamus acts as the primary circadian pacemaker, synchronizing internal functions with external environmental cues, particularly light. This synchronization is essential for good performance and well-being.

The body's internal clock, also known as the circadian clock, regulates sleep-wake cycles, hormone synthesis, body temperature, and metabolism. Circadian rhythms serve an important function in maintaining homeostasis and adapting to environmental changes. The circadian system is mostly influenced by light, particularly natural sunshine. The eyes, particularly the specialized retinal ganglion cells carrying melanopsin, respond to light and send signals to the SCN. This complex signaling process permits the circadian system to align with the

24-hour day-night cycle, guaranteeing proper functioning and synchronization of many physiological activities.

The significance of light in regulating circadian rhythms:

Light exposure, especially in the morning, is critical for synchronizing the circadian clock and sustaining a healthy sleep-wake cycle. Circadian entrainment's effectiveness is influenced by the quality, intensity, and duration of light exposure. Natural sunlight, with its whole range of wavelengths, is particularly effective in controlling circadian cycles. Artificial lighting, such as light-emitting diodes (LEDs), can be designed to mimic the natural light spectrum. Proper light exposure aids in the establishment of a predictable sleep-wake cycle, increase attentiveness during waking hours, and promotes overall well-being.

Circadian rhythm disturbances, such as those produced by irregular light exposure, can result in circadian misalignment.

This misalignment has been linked to a variety of health concerns, including sleep disorders, mood swings, and metabolic abnormalities. Modern lives, which include more indoor time and exposure to artificial light at odd hours, make it difficult to maintain a healthy circadian rhythm. Light therapy, which involves deliberate exposure to bright light, has developed as a therapeutic strategy for circadian rhythm disorders and overall wellness.

<u>Melatonin & Sleep:</u>

Melatonin, also known as the "sleep hormone," is a fundamental regulator of the sleep-wake cycle and is strongly related to circadian rhythms.

Melatonin is synthesized and released by the pineal gland in reaction to darkness, and its levels normally rise in the evening, increasing tiredness and preparing the body for sleep. Light, particularly blue light, decreases melatonin production, signaling the body to wake up. This precise balance of light and darkness affects the quality and timing of sleep.

Understanding the relationship between light and melatonin is critical in treating sleep problems and improving sleep hygiene. Individuals who are exposed to insufficient or irregular light, particularly in the evening, may experience disturbances in melatonin production, resulting in difficulty falling asleep or maintaining a normal sleep pattern. Light therapy, specifically timed exposure to bright light, has been used to modulate melatonin secretion and improve sleep quality. Practitioners seek to restore the natural circadian rhythm and encourage healthy sleep patterns by carefully controlling the timing and intensity of light exposure.

Effects on Mood and Mental Health

Light therapy has a substantial impact on mood and mental health in addition to circadian rhythm modulation and sleep management. Natural light, particularly sunlight, has been linked to greater mood, less depressive symptoms, and a higher sense of well-being. The complex interaction between light and mood is controlled by several neurotransmitters and hormones, including serotonin and dopamine.

Insufficient exposure to natural light, which is common in those who have restricted outside activities or live in areas with little sunlight, has been linked to diseases including seasonal affective disorder (SAD). SAD is defined by recurrent episodes of depression, which often occur during the fall and winter months when daylight hours are reduced. Light therapy, often provided through bright light boxes, is a well-known treatment for SAD. Exposure to intense light replicates the benefits of natural sunlight, which improves mood and alleviates depression symptoms.

Aside from SAD, light therapy has shown potential in treating other mood disorders, such as non-seasonal depression and bipolar disorder. The modulation of neurotransmitters, regulation of circadian rhythms, and influence on sleep patterns all contribute to light's therapeutic effects on mood. As researchers continue to investigate the deep neurobiological underpinnings, light therapy remains an effective adjunctive or independent intervention for those suffering from mood disorders.

Light's Effect on Hormones and Physiology:

Light has a significant impact on the endocrine system and other physiological processes in addition to circadian rhythms and sleep. The complex interaction between light and hormones like cortisol and insulin emphasizes the role of light in metabolic health. Cortisol, also known as the "stress hormone," has a diurnal cycle, increasing in the early morning to promote wakefulness and gradually decreasing towards the evening to aid sleep.

Proper exposure to natural light, particularly in the morning, helps control cortisol levels, promoting a healthy stress response and overall well-being. Disrupted light exposure, on the other hand, might cause cortisol secretion to be dysregulated, potentially contributing to chronic stress and related health consequences. Light therapy, which aligns circadian rhythms and optimizes cortisol secretion, has been investigated as a non-pharmacological solution to stress-related diseases.

Light also regulates insulin sensitivity and glucose metabolism. Studies have shown that strong light, especially in the morning, can enhance insulin sensitivity and lower blood glucose levels.

This effect is attributable to the synchronization of circadian rhythms, which have been linked to metabolic diseases like obesity and type 2 diabetes. Light therapy, with its impact on circadian regulation and hormonal balance, shows promise as a supplementary technique for controlling metabolic illnesses and maintaining general metabolic health.

Light has a wide range of biological impacts, including circadian rhythm regulation, sleep-wake cycle modulation, impact on mood and mental health, and influence on hormones and physiology. The complex interaction between light and the body's internal functions emphasizes the need to keep a healthy relationship with the natural light-dark cycle. Light therapy, which involves strategic exposure to bright light, appears as a versatile and non-invasive intervention that has the potential to address a wide range of health conditions, including sleep difficulties, mood abnormalities, and metabolic disorders. As our understanding of the complex interplay between light and biology grows, the therapeutic uses of light therapy are likely to expand, opening up new pathways for improving human health and well-being.

CHAPTER 3
TYPES OF LIGHT THERAPY

Light therapy, often known as phototherapy, is a medical treatment that uses precise wavelengths of light to cure a variety of ailments. This treatment technique has gained popularity due to its noninvasive nature and capacity to impact biological processes at the cellular level. Several types of light treatment have been developed, each with its unique properties and applications.

Broad-Spectrum Light Therapy

Broad Spectrum Light Therapy uses a wide range of wavelengths from the electromagnetic spectrum, including visible and infrared light. This holistic technique stimulates a variety of cellular processes and is commonly used to treat mood disorders, sleep difficulties, and skin diseases. Because of its adaptability, broad-spectrum light therapy is an effective tool for treating a wide range of health concerns.

<u>Narrowband UVB Therapy.</u>

Narrowband UVB Therapy uses ultraviolet B (UVB) radiation with a restricted wavelength range. This type of light treatment is especially useful for treating skin conditions including psoriasis and vitiligo. Controlled exposure to UVB radiation helps to modify the immunological response and promotes skin cell renewal. Despite its usefulness, caution is advised to reduce the danger of overexposure and potential negative effects from UV radiation.

<u>Blue Light Therapy</u>

Blue Light Therapy focuses on a specific range of the visible light spectrum, primarily wavelengths between 405 and 470 nanometers. This sort of light therapy has been used to treat acne, sleep difficulties, and specific mood disorders. Blue light's antibacterial characteristics make it beneficial in lowering acne-related inflammation, and its influence on circadian cycles helps manage sleep disturbances.

<u>Red Light Therapy</u>

Red Light treatment, also known as low-level laser treatment (LLLT) or photo biomodulation, uses red or near-infrared light with wavelengths ranging from 630 to 850 nanometres. This type of light treatment is effective for wound healing, tissue restoration, and inflammation reduction. Red light's capacity to penetrate deeper into tissues makes it ideal for use in musculoskeletal problems, boosting cellular repair and regeneration.

Green Light Therapy

Green Light Therapy works within the visible light spectrum, focusing on wavelengths between 520 and 550 nanometers. While green light is less often utilized than other types of light therapy, it has shown potential in treating chronic pain and migraine headaches.

Its possible analgesic effects are hypothesized to be connected to neurotransmitter action and pain perception regulation.

Bright Light Therapy

Bright Light Therapy is characterized by the use of high-intensity light, which is typically similar to natural sunlight.

This medication is frequently used to treat illnesses involving circadian rhythm abnormalities, such as seasonal affective disorder (SAD) and sleep difficulties. Bright light helps regulate melatonin production and reset the internal body clock, which contributes to better mood and sleep habits.

<u>Pulsed Light Therapy</u>

Pulsed Light Therapy (PLT), also known as intense pulsed light (IPL), uses short bursts of high-intensity light to treat certain skin disorders such as pigmentation abnormalities and vascular lesions.

The pulsed nature of the light allows for the selective targeting of specific chromophores in the skin, resulting in less damage to nearby tissues.

This method has gained favor in cosmetic dermatology because of its ability to handle a wide range of skin issues.

Infrared Light Therapy

Infrared Light Therapy is the use of light with longer wavelengths than visible light, typically 700 to 1000 nanometers.

This type of therapy penetrates deeper into tissues and is used for a variety of therapeutic goals, such as pain relief, wound healing, and inflammation reduction. Infrared light stimulates cellular processes, causing vasodilation, enhanced circulation, and cellular repair.

The various methods of light treatment show the adaptability and potential of this non-invasive medicinal approach. From treating skin problems to altering mood and circadian rhythms, light therapy is becoming an increasingly essential tool in the healthcare scene. Ongoing research and technology breakthroughs help to increase our understanding and applications of light therapy in boosting general well-being.

CHAPTER 4
APPLICATION OF LIGHT THERAPY

Light therapy, commonly known as phototherapy, is a therapeutic strategy that uses certain wavelengths of light to treat a variety of medical ailments and enhance general health. Light therapy has numerous applications, ranging from mental health to dermatology, demonstrating its adaptability in addressing a variety of health concerns. In this in-depth discussion, we will delve into the nuances of light therapy, including its applications in Seasonal Affective Disorder (SAD), sleep disorders, photodynamic therapy in medicine, skin conditions (specifically acne and psoriasis), psychological and emotional disorders, and sports and performance.

Light therapy for Seasonal Affective Disorder (SAD) represents a significant development in the treatment of mood disorders caused by seasonal variations, particularly the reduction in natural sunlight throughout the fall and winter. SAD symptoms include depression, exhaustion, and abnormalities in sleep patterns. The core premise of light treatment for SAD is to expose patients to bright light that resembles natural sunlight, which regulates circadian cycles and influences neurotransmitter levels. Light treatment has been shown in studies to significantly alleviate SAD symptoms by increasing serotonin and melatonin levels, which contributes to mood stabilization. This therapeutic method has gained popularity as a non-pharmacological and well-tolerated treatment for people who experience seasonal mood swings.

In the field of sleep disorders, light therapy is emerging as a viable technique for regulating circadian rhythms and improving overall sleep quality. Circadian rhythms are critical in regulating the sleep-wake cycle and disrupting them can result in sleep problems. Light treatment, particularly dawn simulation or exposure to strong light in the morning, can help synchronize circadian rhythms, resulting in improved sleep. This use of light therapy includes diseases like insomnia and delayed sleep phase syndrome. Light therapy helps to control sleep-related difficulties by modifying melatonin production and increasing alertness, making it a non-invasive and effective treatment option.

Photodynamic therapy (PDT) is a novel application of light therapy in medicine that involves the use of photosensitizing chemicals activated by certain wavelengths of light to treat various illnesses. PDT involves administering a photosensitiser to the patient, which, when exposed to light of a specific wavelength, releases reactive oxygen species that specifically target and destroy aberrant cells or bacteria. This tailored technique makes PDT useful in the treatment of some malignancies, precancerous lesions, and microbial infections. PDT is an emerging field of study with prospective uses in dermatology, cancer, and antimicrobial therapy, indicating its versatility in medicinal interventions.

Light therapy has been used in dermatology to treat skin disorders such as acne and psoriasis, and it has proven to be beneficial. Blue light therapy is used to treat acne by targeting the germs that cause breakouts, lowering inflammation, and boosting skin repair.

This non-invasive technique has grown in favor of an alternate or complementary treatment for acne, particularly in circumstances when traditional medications are not well accepted. Similarly, phototherapy for psoriasis, a chronic skin disorder characterized by aberrant cell growth, uses tailored ultraviolet (UV) light exposure.

UVB and UVA rays are commonly used to treat psoriasis, slowing skin cell proliferation and alleviating symptoms. The controlled use of light therapy in dermatological disorders highlights its importance as a helpful supplement to conventional treatments, providing patients with alternative options with fewer side effects.

Light therapy appears to be a promising supplementary treatment for illnesses such as depression, anxiety, and bipolar disorder. Light has a direct impact on neurotransmitter modulation and circadian rhythms, which affect mood and emotional well-being. Light treatment for depression, for example, is exposure to strong light that simulates natural sunlight, resulting in higher serotonin levels and a better mood. Light therapy's antidepressant benefits make it a feasible choice for those who do not respond well to typical pharmacological therapies, as well as a supplementary therapy to improve treatment outcomes. Furthermore, evidence suggests that light treatment may have anxiolytic properties, offering a non-pharmacological method for controlling anxiety disorders.

The application of light therapy in sports and performance is an innovative technique for improving athletic performance, circadian rhythm synchronization, and recovery. Jet lag, irregular schedules, and interruptions to their natural circadian cycles are common issues for athletes, and they can all influence performance. Light therapy therapies, such as selective exposure to bright light at specified times, can aid in the regulation of the circadian clock and improve sleep quality, enhancing athletic performance. Furthermore, light treatment may help with the recovery process by altering elements including inflammation and muscular discomfort. As sports science continues to investigate novel tactics for athlete well-being, light therapy emerges as a promising tool for improving both the physical and mental aspects of athletic performance.

The numerous applications of light therapy demonstrate its versatility as a non-invasive and well-tolerated therapeutic intervention. Light therapy is still a topic of active study and therapeutic exploration, with applications ranging from mood disorders and sleep problems to skin ailments, psychological illnesses, and sports performance optimization. As our understanding of the molecular mechanisms underpinning light therapy advances, its potential uses in a variety of medical fields are likely to expand, opening up new possibilities for enhancing patient outcomes and general well-being.

CHAPTER 5
DEVICES AND EQUIPMENT

Light therapy, often known as phototherapy, refers to a range of techniques and equipment used to harness the therapeutic power of light for medical and psychological objectives.

One of the most basic tools in light therapy is the light box, which generates precise wavelengths of light to replicate natural sunlight. Light boxes are often used to treat diseases such as seasonal affective disorder (SAD), a type of depression that occurs annually, usually during the winter when sunshine exposure is limited. These boxes emit strong white light, frequently surpassing 10,000 lux, which stimulates serotonin production and regulates circadian rhythms.

Beyond classic light boxes, LED therapy gadgets have gained popularity in recent years. LEDs emit light in certain colors and wavelengths, enabling for tailored therapy. Different colors are thought to have distinct impacts on the body and mind, with blue light commonly used to treat sleep issues and red light for skin conditions. LED therapy devices are adaptable and may be included in a variety of treatment regimens due to their variable settings.

Laser treatment devices are another type of light therapy that involves the use of coherent and concentrated light to enhance cellular activity. Low-level laser therapy (LLLT) has been studied for its ability to promote tissue healing, reduce inflammation, and alleviate pain. This type of light treatment operates at a lower intensity than surgical lasers, making it appropriate for a variety of medical applications, including wound healing and musculoskeletal disorders.

Wearable light treatment elevates the concept of mobility by allowing individuals to include light therapy in their regular routines. Wearable technologies, such as masks or spectacles, provide tailored light exposure directly to the eyes or skin. This invention not only makes light therapy sessions more convenient but also encourages adherence to treatment plans, which is crucial to their efficacy.

Ensuring the safe use of light treatment devices is critical, which leads us to safety measures and guidelines. As with any medical intervention, there are hazards connected with inappropriate use or prolonged exposure to light. Eye protection is especially important while working with instruments that emit high-intensity light or lasers. Additionally, recognizing the optimal time and intensity of light exposure is critical to avoiding negative consequences. Light therapy professionals emphasize the need for tailored treatment regimens that consider aspects such as skin type, medical history, and the specific ailment being treated.

The variety of devices and equipment used in light therapy reflects our growing understanding of light's healing properties. From the conventional lightbox to cutting-edge wearable gadgets, each instrument has a distinct purpose in treating a variety of medical and psychological issues. As the area evolves, continuous research and technology breakthroughs are likely to help improve and develop ever more complex light treatment systems.

<u>LED Therapy Devices:</u>

LED therapy devices, which use light-emitting diodes to deliver precise wavelengths of light, have emerged as an adaptable and promising technique in the field of light therapy.

The essential premise underlying LED therapy is that different hues of light trigger different physiological responses. Blue light, for example, has been related to better sleep patterns and mood control, whilst red light is commonly used for its potential benefits in skin renewal and wound healing.

One of the key benefits of LED therapy devices is their tunability. Practitioners can pick and deliver specific wavelengths according to the desired therapeutic outcome.

This adaptability allows for the modification of treatment protocols for a wide range of illnesses, including sleep difficulties and dermatological issues. Furthermore, LED gadgets are typically regarded as safe, with minimal danger of side effects when used within specified settings.

Blue light exposure has garnered interest in the context of sleep problems due to its function in circadian rhythm regulation. The human body's internal clock, which is impacted by exposure to natural light, regulates the sleep-wake cycle. Blue light, like the natural light spectrum, decreases melatonin production, increasing wakefulness and alertness during the day. As a result, blue light-emitting LED devices have been used in therapies for insomnia and circadian rhythm sleep problems.

In dermatology, red light therapy with LEDs has shown potential for a variety of skin disorders. Red light has several therapeutic effects, including enhanced collagen formation, improved blood circulation, and decreased inflammation. These advantages make red light therapy an important tool in the treatment of acne, wrinkles, and wound healing. LED devices built for skincare applications frequently include various colors, allowing practitioners to combine wavelengths for more thorough treatment regimens.

Despite the benefits of LED therapy, it is critical to evaluate the possible downsides and restrictions. The efficacy of LED treatment can vary depending on the individual ailment being treated, the wavelength used, and the time of exposure. Individual responses to light therapy can also vary, needing a specific treatment plan.

Ongoing research on the subject seeks to identify ideal settings for LED therapy across a variety of applications, hence contributing to the refining of therapeutic protocols.

LED therapy devices are a versatile and adaptable instrument in the field of light therapy. Their capacity to produce specific wavelengths opens up possibilities for a wide range of applications, including sleep management and dermatological therapies. As research uncovers the complexities of light's effect on the body, LED therapy is positioned to play an increasingly important part in the changing landscape of therapeutic techniques.

Laser Therapy Devices:

Laser treatment devices, which exploit the special features of focused and coherent light, are a separate category within the larger field of light therapy. Low-level laser treatment (LLLT), often called cold laser therapy, uses low-intensity lasers or light-emitting diodes to boost cellular function. Unlike surgical lasers used for cutting or ablation, LLLT operates at low power levels and produces little heat, making it ideal for therapeutic purposes.

One of the fundamental principles of laser therapy is photo biomodulation, which occurs when light energy is absorbed by cellular components, resulting in biochemical changes. These changes may include higher ATP synthesis, improved cellular metabolism, and the release of signaling molecules that aid in tissue repair and anti-inflammatory responses. As a result, laser treatment has found applications in a wide range of medical sectors, including musculoskeletal problems and wound healing.

Laser therapy is effective in the treatment of musculoskeletal problems by relieving pain and stimulating tissue repair.

The precise application of laser light to wounded or inflamed tissues is thought to regulate biological processes, resulting in reduced pain perception and faster recovery. Conditions such as osteoarthritis, tendinopathy, and sports injuries have been studied for the possible benefits of laser therapy.

Wound healing is another area where laser therapy devices have demonstrated promise. Laser therapy promotes cellular proliferation and angiogenesis, which aids in tissue regeneration.

The anti-inflammatory properties of LLLT aid in the healing process, making it an important tool in the treatment of chronic wounds, ulcers, and post-surgical recovery.

Despite the expanding body of research demonstrating laser therapy's therapeutic potential, there are several limitations and caveats. The ideal therapeutic parameters, including wavelength and dosage, are still being researched. Furthermore, individual responses to laser therapy may differ, necessitating a tailored approach to treatment planning. Safety factors, such as the risk of eye damage from high-power lasers, highlight the need to follow established rules and regulations.

Laser therapy devices provide a novel and tailored method for harnessing the healing power of light. The modality's efficacy and safety are being investigated in a variety of settings, including musculoskeletal applications and wound healing. As research progresses, new insights into the molecular mechanisms of photo biomodulation are anticipated to influence the refinement and expansion of laser treatment in clinical practice.

<u>Wearable light therapy:</u>

Wearable light treatment is a game changer in the field of phototherapy, allowing people to easily incorporate light-based interventions into their daily lives. Wearable devices' mobility and convenience overcome some of the constraints of traditional light treatment techniques, increasing user adherence and broadening the variety of illnesses that can be effectively treated.

One popular type of wearable light therapy gadget is the light therapy mask. These masks typically cover the eyes and provide controlled light exposure to stimulate photoreceptors in the retina. Wearable masks can alter circadian rhythms by directly influencing the eyes, making them useful tools for treating sleep disorders and other illnesses characterized by interrupted sleep-wake cycles.

These masks' designs frequently include features like adjustable light intensity and changeable wavelength choices.

Wearable light therapy can also take the form of glasses-style gadgets. These devices, which resemble traditional eyewear, are equipped with light-emitting elements that direct therapeutic light to the eyes. The design improves user comfort and practicality, allowing people to engage in light treatment while doing a variety of tasks. Wearable light therapy glasses are commonly used to treat illnesses like seasonal affective disorder (SAD) and circadian rhythm abnormalities.

The use of wearable light treatment in daily activities goes beyond ocular applications. Devices designed for skin interventions, such as wearable LED patches or bands, provide tailored exposure to specific body locations. This breakthrough is especially important in dermatology, where light treatment has shown promise in treating acne, psoriasis, and skin aging. The convenience of wearable devices increases patient compliance, which is crucial to the efficacy of long-term therapeutic approaches.

Despite the benefits of wearable light treatment, user comfort, device ergonomics, and safety remain critical. To ensure user acceptance and adherence, devices must be designed to minimize discomfort while providing effective light exposure. Furthermore, instructions for safe usage, such as recommended durations and intensity levels, must be properly communicated to users to avoid potential negative consequences.

Wearable light treatment marks a significant breakthrough in the accessibility and incorporation of phototherapy into daily life. Wearable devices provide a fresh technique for delivering focused light exposure, with applications ranging from sleep disorders to dermatological issues. As technology advances, wearable light treatment devices are anticipated to play an important role in the changing landscape of tailored and convenient therapeutic interventions.

<u>Safety precautions and guidelines:</u>

The safe and successful use of light therapy equipment requires a thorough grasp of safety considerations and guidelines to reduce potential dangers. As with any medical intervention, striking a balance between therapeutic advantages and avoiding negative consequences is critical. Safety issues in light therapy include a variety of factors such as device-specific precautions, exposure length and intensity, and personalized treatment programs.

Lightboxes, which are widely employed in the treatment of illnesses such as seasonal affective disorder (SAD), necessitate careful consideration of exposure settings. While these gadgets emit bright, white light to resemble sunlight, care must be taken to avoid damaging the eyes and skin. Eye protection, in the form of UV-blocking goggles, is frequently recommended to protect the eyes from potential harm, particularly when working with bright light. The duration and timing of light exposure are crucial elements, and guidelines normally indicate suggested daily durations and treatment times.

LED therapy devices, which are noted for their adaptability and configurable settings, necessitate adherence to safety guidelines.

The wavelengths and intensities chosen should be based on the desired therapeutic effect, taking into account parameters such as skin type and the ailment being treated. Individual responses must be properly monitored and prescribed exposure times followed. In dermatological applications, where LED devices are used for skin rejuvenation or acne treatment, keeping the device clean and well-maintained is critical to avoiding infections or skin irritation.

Laser therapy equipment, although providing precise and focused treatment, necessitates strict adherence to safety protocols. The risk of eye damage mandates the use of protective eyewear intended to block the laser's precise wavelengths. Setting proper dose parameters, such as wavelength and energy levels, is critical for improving therapeutic outcomes while reducing hazards. Laser treatment professionals must be trained to operate the devices safely and properly.

Wearable light therapy systems, while developed for user comfort, must also emphasize safety. Wearable gadgets are safer to use when they are designed to be comfortable, follow ergonomic principles, and have clear user instructions. In ocular applications, such as light therapy masks or spectacles, it is critical to ensure that the devices do not cause eye discomfort or pressure. Guidelines for regular cleaning and maintenance of wearable gadgets help them last longer and prevent hygiene issues.

The safe implementation of light therapy necessitates a complex strategy that includes device-specific safeguards, personalized treatment plans, and strict adherence to established norms. As the sector advances, continuing research and collaboration among healthcare experts and device makers will help to build uniform safety measures. Prioritizing safety in the use of light therapy devices ensures that therapeutic advantages are maximized while bad effects are minimized, promoting trust in the efficacy of these treatments.

CHAPTER 6
RESEARCH AND CLINICAL STUDIES

Scientific research on the efficacy of light therapy:

Light treatment, commonly known as phototherapy, has been extensively researched for its effectiveness in treating a variety of diseases, including mood disorders and sleep difficulties. Numerous scientific research have investigated the mechanics underlying light therapy and its effects on human physiology. One significant field of research is the treatment of seasonal affective disorder (SAD), a kind of depression that occurs primarily during the winter months when natural sunlight exposure is limited. Studies have repeatedly demonstrated that exposure to strong light, particularly in the morning, can help with SAD symptoms by regulating circadian rhythms and modulating neurotransmitter levels. Furthermore, studies have looked into the efficacy of light therapy in treating various mood disorders such as major depressive disorder (MDD) and bipolar disorder. The findings imply that light therapy could be a useful supplementary treatment, particularly in circumstances when standard therapies are ineffective.

Beyond mood problems, light therapy has shown promise in treating sleep-related ailments. According to research, exposure to specific wavelengths of light can influence the generation of melatonin, a hormone that regulates sleep-wake cycles. This has resulted in the creation of light therapy interventions for ailments such as sleeplessness and circadian rhythm problems.

Furthermore, research has looked into the possibilities of light therapy in treating non-psychiatric illnesses including psoriasis. The underlying assumption is that certain light wavelengths can alter biological processes, resulting in therapeutic effects across multiple medical areas.

However, the limited literature on light therapy must be thoroughly evaluated. While several researches found good results, there are differences in methodology, sample sizes, and end measures. Some studies have also emphasized the necessity of taking individual characteristics into account while responding to light therapy, underlining the need for tailored treatment techniques.

Furthermore, the duration and intensity of light exposure, as well as the timing of sessions, have been recognized as important influences on treatment outcomes. As the field evolves, current research strives to improve protocols, standardize processes, and better understand the complex impacts of light therapy on different groups.

<u>Ongoing Research and Future Directions:</u>

As light therapy develops popularity in medical and psychological interventions, current research aims to broaden our understanding and explore new applications. One significant field of research is the neurobiological mechanisms by which light affects mood and cognition. Advanced neuroimaging techniques, such as functional magnetic resonance imaging (fMRI) and positron emission tomography (PET), allow researchers to investigate changes in brain activity and neurotransmitter levels in response to light exposure. This neuroscientific method advances our understanding of the brain circuits involved in the therapeutic benefits of light therapy, potentially paving the door for more focused therapies.

Another area of ongoing study is on improving light therapy methods. Researchers are experimenting with varied light intensities, durations, and spectrum compositions to find the most efficient parameters for various circumstances. This includes researching the possible benefits of employing specific wavelengths of light and designing personalized treatment strategies based on unique patient characteristics.

Furthermore, technological improvements have resulted in the creation of wearable light gadgets and smart lighting systems, making light therapy more flexible and comfortable in everyday life.

Light therapy's inclusion into interdisciplinary therapeutic techniques is currently under investigation. A collaborative study involving psychiatrists, psychologists, sleep specialists, and other healthcare professionals seeks to determine the synergistic benefits of combining light therapy with pharmaceutical and psychotherapy therapies. Such comprehensive approaches may improve treatment outcomes and provide more holistic answers for people dealing with complex mental health disorders.

Beyond therapeutic uses, researchers are investigating the potential of light therapy to improve cognitive performance and mitigate the effects of shift work and jet lag. Investigations investigating the impact of light on non-visual functions, such as alertness and attention, help to design solutions for people who work in demanding conditions or have disrupted sleep-wake cycles.

While most current research focuses on the benefits of light treatment, continuing studies also address potential side effects and safety concerns. Understanding the limitations and hazards associated with light therapy is critical for its appropriate and effective use in a variety of populations.

<u>Limitations and Challenges of Light Therapy Research</u>:

Despite promising discoveries and growing acceptance of light therapy as a treatment technique, there remain significant limits and problems in the present body of evidence.

One overriding problem is the variability of study designs and methodology, which makes it difficult to compare and generalize results from diverse investigations. Standardizing protocols for light treatment studies is a difficult endeavor due to differences in equipment, doses, and participant characteristics.

Another important concern is the placebo effect, which can have a considerable impact on the results of light treatment studies. Participants may report increases in mood or sleep simply because they believe the treatment is helpful, making it difficult to isolate the precise effects of light exposure. This underlines the need to use strict control conditions and blinded trial designs to reduce placebo effects.

The longevity of therapeutic effects, as well as the possibility of relapse after discontinuing light therapy, present additional concerns. Some studies indicate that the advantages of light therapy may be transitory, necessitating continuous or maintenance treatment to maintain therapeutic effects. Understanding the long-term ramifications and establishing ways to prevent relapse is critical for improving treatment outcomes.

Individual variability in responsiveness to light treatment is a complex issue that researchers are actively tackling. Age, gender, genetics, and baseline symptom intensity all have an impact on how people respond to light exposure.

Treatment protocols must be tailored to account for individual differences, which necessitates a customized medicine approach that takes into consideration a variety of biological and behavioral aspects.

Safety concerns are also important to consider while using light therapy. While it is generally regarded safe when used carefully, potential adverse effects include eye strain, headaches, and worsening of pre-existing problems. The parameters for safe and successful light treatment, including ideal light intensity, duration, and timing, are currently being researched.

While light therapy shows great promise as a non-invasive and well-tolerated treatment for a variety of conditions, more research is needed to fine-tune protocols, gain a better understanding of underlying mechanisms, and address the complexities of individual variability and safety concerns.

The interdisciplinary character of current research reflects light therapy's dynamic evolution as a vital tool in the larger landscape of healthcare interventions. As the field evolves, a collaborative and evidence-based approach will be critical to realizing light therapy's full promise for varied patient populations.

CHAPTER 7
IMPLEMENTATION AND BEST PRACTICES

Choosing the Proper Light Therapy Approach

Choosing the right light therapy strategy is a critical step toward ensuring its effectiveness. Different situations necessitate distinct wavelengths, intensities, and periods of light exposure. For example, Seasonal Affective Disorder (SAD) frequently reacts well to bright light with a color temperature of 5,000 to 10,000 lux, but circadian rhythm disorders may benefit from lower-intensity light exposure in the morning or evening. Understanding the subtleties of each ailment and adapting light treatment accordingly is critical for successful results. When deciding on the best light therapy strategy, both clinicians and individuals must evaluate the patient's sensitivity to light, medical history, and the specific symptoms being addressed.

Setting Up An Effective Light Therapy Space

Creating an environment suitable for light therapy is critical to its success. Proper setup entails placing the light source at the proper angle and distance, usually within two feet of the individual. The light box should produce the specified lux level and be aimed at the eyes without causing pain. Furthermore, reducing glare and maintaining constant daily exposure is critical. Adequate ventilation and comfy sitting help to provide a favorable therapeutic experience. Professionals must educate individuals on the need to stick to a consistent schedule and follow the prescribed setup requirements to maximize the therapeutic effects of light therapy.

Furthermore, focusing on the aesthetics and utility of the place can improve overall compliance and user experience.

<u>Duration and Timing Guidelines</u>

Determining the optimal duration and timing of light therapy sessions necessitates a thorough understanding of circadian cycles and treatment objectives. Individuals should start with shorter sessions, typically 20-30 minutes, and gradually increase exposure if well tolerated. The timing of light exposure is critical for regulating circadian rhythms; morning light is frequently advised for insomnia or delayed sleep phase syndrome, but evening light exposure may benefit advanced sleep phase syndrome. Finding the appropriate balance between duration and timing is critical for avoiding unwanted adverse effects and maximizing therapeutic benefits. Clinicians should take into account individual variations in light sensitivity and adapt duration and timing recommendations accordingly, emphasizing the significance of consistency for long-term favorable results.

Integrating Light Therapy into Everyday Life

Integrating light therapy into daily routines demands a deliberate and individualized approach. Professionals must educate people on the value of consistency and sticking to a set routine. Creating techniques to effortlessly integrate light treatment into daily life, such as introducing it into morning routines or work surroundings, can help increase compliance. Behavioral therapies, such as habit-building and positive reinforcement, can be used to encourage long-term compliance. Individual lifestyle aspects, such as work schedules and personal preferences, must also be considered when integrating light therapy. Collaboration between healthcare practitioners and individuals can help to build practical and long-term strategies for integrating light therapy into daily life.

Combining Light Therapy and Other Treatments

In many circumstances, light therapy is used in conjunction with a full therapeutic strategy rather than as a stand-alone treatment. Understanding the synergies and potential conflicts between light therapy and other therapies is critical for increasing benefits while reducing dangers. For example, combining light therapy and medicine for depression may improve treatment efficacy, but potential interactions and adverse effects must be carefully examined. Communication and collaboration among healthcare practitioners managing various elements of therapy are critical to ensuring a comprehensive and coordinated approach. Clinicians should evaluate the individual's complete treatment plan, including drugs, psychotherapy, and lifestyle modifications, to build an integrated and harmonious approach that addresses the varied nature of diverse diseases.

The proper implementation of light therapy necessitates a thorough understanding and application of many ideas. Choosing the correct light treatment strategy necessitates consideration of individual diseases and symptoms while creating an effective light therapy area necessitates meticulous attention to detail in terms of posture, comfort, and appearance. Individual circadian cycles and therapeutic goals must be considered when developing duration and timing guidelines, with a focus on consistency for best results. Integrating light therapy into daily life requires a targeted and planned approach to promote adherence and habit formation. Finally, combining light therapy with other therapies necessitates careful planning to optimize therapeutic benefits while minimizing potential conflicts. A thorough understanding and use of these concepts contribute to light therapy's success as a useful intervention in a variety of clinical and therapeutic settings.

CHAPTER 8
SUCCESS STORIES AND TESTIMONIALS

Light treatment, often known as phototherapy or heliotherapy, has received widespread attention and recognition for its potential to heal a variety of illnesses. One intriguing component of the discussion surrounding light therapy is the abundance of success stories and testimonials offered by people who have tried this therapeutic intervention. These accounts offer essential insights into the subjective sensations and reported benefits of light therapy. One recurring element in personal testimonies is the good influence on mood disorders like Seasonal Affective Disorder (SAD) and depression. Individuals frequently report a considerable improvement in their overall well-being, which some attribute to the management of circadian rhythms and increased serotonin production.

These anecdotal findings not only demonstrate the potential usefulness of light treatment but also highlight the necessity for additional scientific research to validate and comprehend these subjective outcomes.

Personal Experiences With Light Therapy:

Personal experiences with light therapy include a wide spectrum of health conditions, giving light to its many applications. Individuals with SAD frequently report a noticeable shift in their mood and energy levels following regular exposure to light treatment lamps. According to reports, the strong light resembles natural sunlight, influencing the creation of melatonin and serotonin, which are important neurotransmitters for mood regulation and sleep-wake cycles. Furthermore, anecdotal evidence goes beyond mood problems, with people reporting their experiences utilizing light therapy for skin conditions such as psoriasis. Some people report relief from symptoms like itching and inflammation, attributing it to the anti-inflammatory properties of certain wavelengths of light. These personal experiences add to the expanding amount of qualitative evidence showing the potential benefit of light therapy in a variety of health contexts.

Case Studies for Successful Light Therapy Interventions:

While personal testimonials give useful information, case studies provide a more systematic and in-depth look at successful light therapy therapies. These extensive assessments of particular instances enable researchers and doctors to investigate the nuances of how light treatment interacts with specific health issues. Case studies on people suffering from circadian rhythm disorders, for example, show how difficult it is to customize light therapy procedures to synchronize the internal body clock with external environmental cues. Successful outcomes in these circumstances frequently require rigorous adjustments to light exposure duration, intensity, and timing. Similarly, case studies on psychiatric diseases investigate the efficacy of light therapy as an adjuvant or independent treatment. Observations of symptom reduction in people with major depressive illness, bipolar disorder, and insomnia highlight light's therapeutic potential in modifying brain circuits and hormone modulation. These case studies not only help us comprehend light therapy's clinical applications but also open the path for more targeted and tailored interventions.

Exploring success stories and testimonials, as well as thorough case studies, provides a rich tapestry of data supporting the efficacy of light therapy across a wide range of health issues. Personal experiences provide insight into the subjective changes claimed by individuals, whereas case studies provide a more thorough and methodical evaluation of light's therapeutic potential. As we navigate the junction of anecdotal evidence and scientific investigation, it becomes clear that light therapy has potential as a diverse and non-invasive treatment.

However, additional research, such as randomized controlled trials and longitudinal studies, is required to build a strong evidence base and refine the clinical applications of light therapy in mainstream healthcare.

CHAPTER 9
ETHICAL CONSIDERATIONS AND SAFETY

<u>Ethical Applications of Light Therapy:</u>

The ethical use of light therapy includes a variety of factors centered on the appropriate and humane deployment of this treatment approach. Practitioners and researchers working with light therapy must follow ethical norms that stress patient welfare, autonomy, and informed consent. One key issue is ensuring that people who participate in light therapy research or treatments understand the therapy's nature, purpose, and potential outcomes. Informed permission is especially important when working with disadvantaged groups or experimental techniques. Furthermore, practitioners should attempt to maintain confidentiality by respecting patients' privacy and protecting sensitive information about their treatment. The ethical considerations include the appropriate use of placebo controls in research settings, minimizing potential biases, and guaranteeing transparency in reporting results. Upholding the principles of beneficence and nonmaleficence is critical, highlighting the importance of maximizing therapeutic benefits while limiting potential injury or pain to those undergoing light treatment. Furthermore, equity and access issues should be addressed, ensuring that the advantages of light therapy are available to a wide range of populations without perpetuating gaps.

Safety Precautions and Potential Risks:

Ensuring the safety of people receiving light therapy is a critical part of its implementation. Safety considerations require a detailed understanding of the physiological and psychological impacts of light exposure, and practitioners must tailor therapies to specific requirements and situations. One critical factor is establishing the optimum light intensity and duration to avoid negative consequences including eye strain, headaches, and sleep problems. Proper eye protection is essential, particularly while using high-intensity light sources, to reduce the risk of retinal injury. Furthermore, it is critical to examine the possible influence of light treatment on people who have pre-existing diseases such as photosensitive epilepsy or certain skin problems. Practitioners should undertake thorough examinations of individuals' medical histories and work with other healthcare experts to uncover relevant contraindications. Adherence to safety rules, such as the use of standardized equipment and monitoring protocols, is critical in avoiding unexpected consequences. Regular patient monitoring during and after light therapy sessions enables early detection of any adverse effects, allowing for quick intervention and treatment plan adjustments.

<u>Regulatory Standards and Certification:</u>

Light therapy is subject to a variety of regulatory requirements and certifications designed to ensure treatment quality, safety, and efficacy. Regulatory agencies play an important role in developing rules that govern the use of light therapy devices, practitioner qualifications, and clinical study procedures. Compliance with these guidelines is critical for practitioners, researchers, and manufacturers seeking to ensure the legitimacy and reliability of light therapy interventions.

Device certification processes include rigorous testing to check safety features, performance, and compliance with set standards. Practitioners are frequently required to complete specialized training and certification to verify their competency in providing light therapy safely and successfully. Regulatory agencies also monitor ongoing research to assess the developing scientific understanding of light treatment and revise guidelines as needed. By complying with regulatory norms, the field of light therapy can develop trust among healthcare professionals, researchers, and the general public, increasing confidence in the therapeutic method and its potential advantages.

CONCLUSION

Light therapy is a diverse and promising therapeutic technique, with a growing body of evidence supporting its usefulness across a wide range of medical disorders. Light therapy has proved its ability to improve people's well-being, from its origins in the treatment of seasonal affective disorder to its uses in dermatology, sleep problems, and beyond. However, like with any therapeutic intervention, ethical considerations, safety measures, and regulatory compliance are critical to its appropriate and effective usage.

Ethically, the use of light therapy requires a dedication to transparency, informed consent, and patient autonomy.

Researchers and practitioners must be aware of potential biases, provide equal access to therapies, and prioritize participants' well-being. Safety considerations include paying close attention to light intensity, duration, and potential contraindications, with an emphasis on avoiding negative consequences and protecting patients' health. The regulatory landscape is critical in developing and maintaining standards for the development, usage, and certification of light therapy equipment, hence increasing the field's reputation and reliability.

Moving forward, continuing study and collaboration among clinicians, researchers, and regulatory agencies will help us better understand the mechanics of light therapy and expand its applicability. Continued attention to ethical principles and safety rules will be critical for mitigating potential dangers and improving the overall quality of care given by light therapy. As the discipline advances, interdisciplinary initiatives will contribute to a thorough understanding of light therapy's various uses, securing its place as a vital and evidence-based tool in the larger landscape of healthcare interventions.

www.ingramcontent.com/pod-product-compliance
Lightning Source LLC
Chambersburg PA
CBHW050650250726
48662CB00002B/593